Going Dry

A WORKBOOK

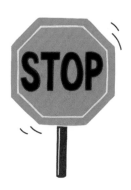 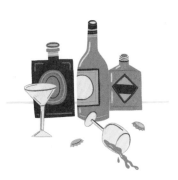 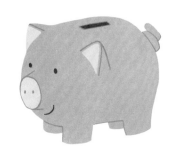

 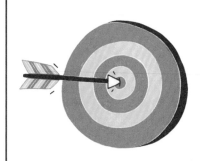 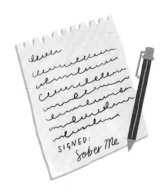

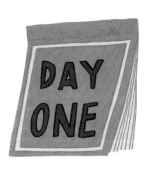 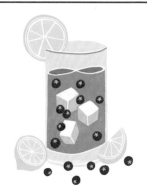 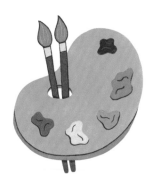

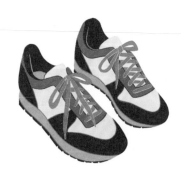 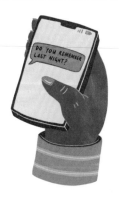 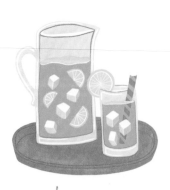

Going Dry

A WORKBOOK

A Practical Guide to Drinking Less and Living More

HILARY SHEINBAUM

Foreword by Lauryn Bosstick

FAIR WINDS

Quarto.com

© 2024 Quarto Publishing Group USA Inc.
Text © 2024 Hilary Sheinbaum

First Published in 2024 by Fair Winds Press,
an imprint of The Quarto Group, 100 Cummings
Center, Suite 265-D, Beverly, MA 01915, USA.
T (978) 282-9590 F (978) 283-2742

Fair Winds Press titles are also available at discount for
retail, wholesale, promotional, and bulk purchase. For de-
tails, contact the Special Sales Manager by email at spe-
cialsales@quarto.com or by mail at The Quarto Group,
Attn: Special Sales Manager, 100 Cummings Center,
Suite 265-D, Beverly, MA 01915, USA.

28 27 26 25 24   1 2 3 4 5

ISBN: 978-0-7603-8852-5

Digital edition published in 2024
eISBN: 978-0-7603-8853-2

Design and Page Layout: Kelley Galbreath
Illustration: Rosie Foden Limited except pages 18,
 104–105 are Shutterstock

Printed in China

Advice and interactive elements within the text, dry
months overall, and dry challenges are not substitutions
or replacements for recovery programs. Please speak with
your doctor if you are struggling with substances.

Dedicated to _you_.
Cheers.

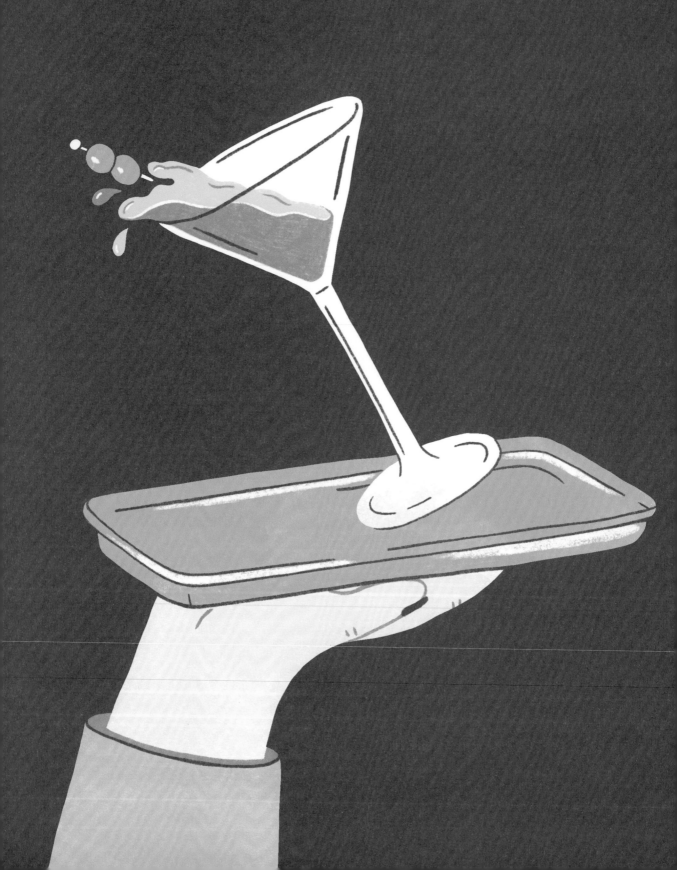

CONTENTS

Foreword

A FEW YEARS AGO, MY HUSBAND AND I decided to go sober for seventy days while committing to a program of meditation and daily movement during that time. To say that it was life-changing is an understatement. Very quickly I had more clarity, focus, peace of mind, muscle tone, better skin, and more energy. What was most surprising to me was how quickly I was able to feel and see those changes. What started as a goal of not drinking for seventy days before an upcoming trip to Cabo San Lucas, Mexico, turned into a total lifestyle shift of movement, mindfulness, and self-care that made going alcohol-free an even bigger priority than it was before. With the money we saved from not going to restaurants and having drinks, we decided to invest in a trainer, sauna, and cold plunge and make it a priority to take care of ourselves FIRST.

The benefits may look different for everyone, but the trickle effects of not drinking alcohol for us are going to bed earlier, waking up earlier, drinking less coffee, having energy for the whole day to work and be present for our kids, more time for reading/meditating/exercising, and being more effective at those things because we aren't canceling them out with cocktails. We still enjoy some drinks once in a while, but we know that for us, there's a time and a place we choose to indulge.

If you're up for a dry challenge, Hilary's exercises in *Going Dry: A Workbook* are an incredible tool to track the changes you feel emotionally and physically. They can help you express how you're feeling, what time of day you're experiencing those feelings, and how you feel before and after you drink alcohol. It's helpful to see your different moods, how you feel after a night involving alcohol or no alcohol, feelings the next morning, and so on. It's very helpful to have this tool in your toolbox when undertaking the journey of sobriety, however long it is.

Next time I cut alcohol I will be referencing Hilary's guide. I usually try to pick three months out of the year to go dry, and I know this tool will upgrade the entire experience.

I highly recommend this workbook to anyone who is sober-curious or who just wants to test out not drinking for a week, month, or year. After all, what's better than giving yourself the gift of clarity, discipline, and extreme awareness all while upgrading your life?

Sincerely,
Lauryn Bosstick, founder of The Skinny Confidential

Introduction

WELCOME TO *GOING DRY: A WORKBOOK*!

Perhaps you're new to this dry lifestyle thing. Or maybe this isn't your first rodeo, but it still feels that way sometimes. Wherever you're coming from, and whatever you're feeling right now—it's all OKAY.

I, for one, am so happy you're here. In case you were wondering: This dry-ish me wasn't always how I operated (in fact, it was quite the opposite—more on that soon). But, at this stage, the lifestyle I live and breathe doesn't feel as alien to me as it did just a few years ago. Even though it's been years since my first Dry January (2017) and I sometimes think I know all there is to know, I still learn and find brand-new, enlightening, fun, empowering, bold, calming, *and* energizing experiences all the time—without drinking.

Giving up or reducing alcohol for a mere month has so many benefits—I mean, *so many*. While nothing is guaranteed in life, some of the changes you'll likely experience include better sleep, clearer skin, improved digestion, financial savings, a clearer mind, more energy, and newfound relationships with the people around you (not to mention an improved relationship with alcohol). What did I miss in my list there? Well, you'll just have to see for yourself . . .

While you're here, I want to mention that the point of this book isn't to reprimand you for drinking—at all. Instead, it's an easy-going, judgment-free companion to help you explore a life without alcohol at any time—during celebrations, during relationships (actual or potential ones with family, friends, and partners), or when you're happy, sad, bored, indifferent, and everything else. Simply put, the exercises in this workbook encourage you to spend your days and nights without consuming adult beverages to see if it suits you for the better.

In this workbook, you'll gather personal insights and reflect on going dry via fun, interactive, and nonjudgmental prompts, puzzles, quizzes, and more. You'll assess where you are now (right this second!) before diving in and explore the potential benefits and your expectations as well as the probable roadblocks standing (or sipping) in your way. Whether you're Type A or never make a set-in-stone promise, this workbook will help you plan ahead for fun, booze-free days and occasional not-so-welcome feedback. And you'll be primed to spot the differences between how you're feeling now, at the beginning of your journey, and how you will feel once you've got a few days or weeks or months under your belt. Finally, after all that, I'll include some pointers and prompts to encourage and support you in sustaining all the good stuff that comes out of this experimental period that you've dedicated to going dry.

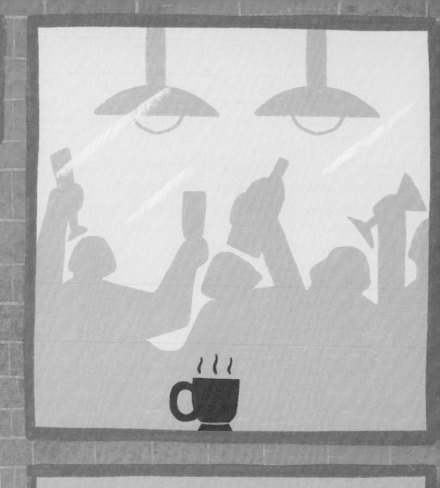

Sound good? Great! But before we get started, why should you even listen to me, right? Here's my super-quick story. My name is Hilary (hi!). The first time I went dry began over a lighthearted bet that I made—with bubbly in hand—on December 31, 2016, just a few minutes before midnight and the start of a new year. At the time it was my literal job as a journalist to cover trends and prominent figures in the wine, beer, spirit, and cocktail space. New bar opening? It was on my radar. New cocktail menu at a restaurant? I was there to report on it. Launch of a new, weird, flavored spirit? I was sipping . . . in the name of research. When I wasn't imbibing for a story, I was on the red carpet interviewing celebrities and attending after-parties with expensive wines and top-shelf liquor. Sometimes drinking on the job was part of the job. Until, on that particular New Year's Eve, I suddenly decided to make a silly wager on a whim. From that moment on, my relationship with drinking changed—at least for the next month.

Will the enclosed exercises upend life as you know it? Not to sound dramatic, but . . . maybe! Whether you choose to give up alcohol for a week(end), a month, six months, a year, or forever, working through the forthcoming prompts, charts, and activities will undoubtedly change something in you—whether that's your sleep, your mood, the way you spend your time, or the way you think about ordering a beverage at a bar or restaurant. A life with less alcohol is different—a little harder in some ways but a lot fuller in others. It's my hope that this book will help you weigh the benefits against the obstacles and discover that different, in this case, definitely means better!

One last thing: I'm not a doctor, so if you have any serious questions or larger concerns about alcohol or your drinking habits or if you are looking for medical guidance, please speak with your physician, who has a degree in that stuff. Advice and interactive elements within the text, dry months overall, and dry challenges are not substitutions or replacements for recovery programs. Please speak with your doctor if you are struggling with substances.

Okay. Now that you know where this is all coming from: Are you ready to go dry?

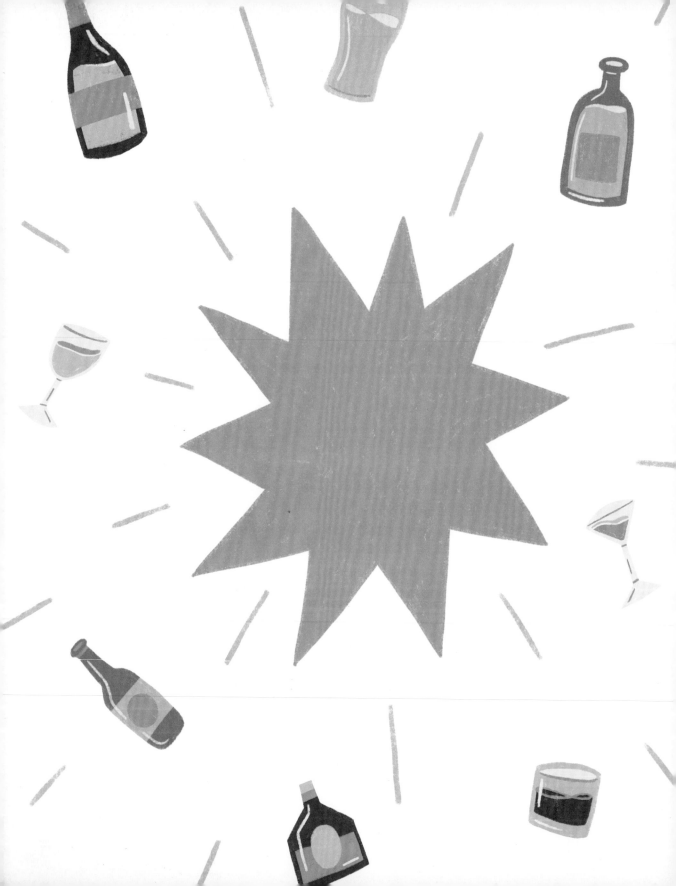

1

Assessing Where You're at Now

ON YOUR MARK, GET SET . . . wait *just* a minute.

I know it's exciting (and sometimes scary) to jump into the start of something new, but before we officially begin, let's get acquainted with you, as you are, right this second.

When I embarked on my first dry month, I went into it totally unprepared. I still had bottles of wine stacked up in my apartment. Looking back on it, I had no guide or idea of what I was doing (or why, besides winning a bet and a gifted meal!).

In my case, I didn't have the time to analyze what I wanted out of going dry that first year. I was curious what it would entail and what positive changes it would bring, but I didn't have any expectations.

Throughout the past couple of years, I've found it incredibly helpful to meet myself where I am. It's been super beneficial to see how my previous experiences have affected my current lifestyle. From my past experiences with going dry, I've been able to envision where I want to be and what I want to gain or learn or seek while I'm going through it. That is what this first chapter is all about. These are the questions, queries, and guided thought processes I wish I'd had that first Dry January so you can get a sense of where you're at and what you want to get out of this process.

You might not have thought about any of this previously (like I said, I didn't!) and you might not want to analyze every. single. detail. But as with everything in this workbook, it's just a suggestion! My recommendation is to complete this section and completely forget about it, then come back later to see if and how things have progressed for you. (That choice is yours, of course! Visit this chapter every damn day if you so choose.)

Ready to get reflective? Let's begin.

Realistic Reasons

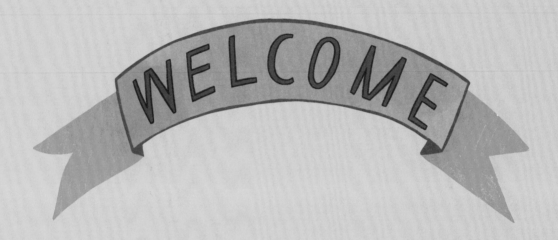

GET OUT YOUR PENS, your colorful markers, and your calligraphy set! (Well, at least one of those things anyway.) Whether a friend gifted you this book, or you were attracted to a colorful new cover in a store or online, or you'd been pondering practical methods for how to start drinking less—welcome! For this first prompt, we're going to talk about what brought you here. Are you looking to do a Dry January, a Sober October, a No-Drink November? Or are you beginning your journey on a random Wednesday? Or maybe it's not about completely going dry and you're just looking to drink a little less? Consider your honest, practical motives for picking up this workbook and fill in your thoughts in the space provided.

Dry Experiences

COME HERE OFTEN? What have your previous experiences with going dry been like? Have you participated in a dry weekend, a dry month, or a dry [insert any period of time here] before? Maybe you've witnessed friends and family take part in dry challenges. Feel free to name-drop those people and discuss their influence here as well. Whether it's your first time going dry or your fifth, what are you looking to get out of consuming less alcohol? It can be anything! Better health and energy or trying something new—write that down here.

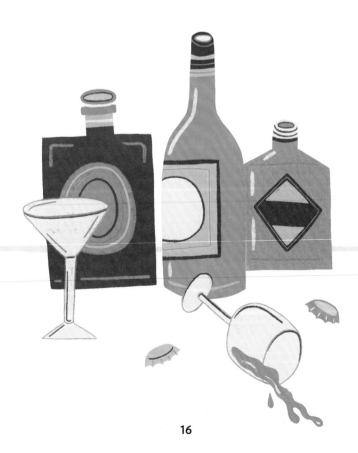

Emoting & Emojis

WHERE ARE YOU TODAY? Okay, not literally, like in London or Paris or New York (but sure, feel free to include that if you want). While your immediate physical environment can influence your drinking or nondrinking habits, we're talking more about your emotional landscape here, as represented by that early twenty-first century icon of emotion: the emoji. The following interactive chart is designed for you to check in on a regular basis and record how you're feeling using a simple emoji to represent your emotional state as you go through your dry journey. Start with today. Come back tomorrow (and the next day and the next). For each day, record the date, an emoji for how you're feeling (you can use one of our suggestions or make up your own), and any notes or details you'd like to include.

DATE	EMOTION (EMOJI)	NOTES
12/2	☺	I felt good because I didn't drink. No hangovers!
12/3	☹	Too many shots, hungover.

What Does Drinking Mean to You?

HOW DO YOU PERCEIVE ALCOHOL? From iconic moments in pop culture to IRL experiences—what is your take on booze? What does it signify when you know alcohol is present or being served at dinner, a celebration, or a random Tuesday, in the home or anywhere else? What feeling—or range of emotions and feelings—do you have toward drinking? Yeah. That's a loaded question. So, take all the time and space you need to write down your thoughts.

_____

_____

_____

_____

_____

_____

_____

_____

_____

Buzzy Words

ON THE NOTE OF PERCEPTION and what drinking means to you, what are some buzz-words (pun intended) that you associate with going dry? For what it's worth, these can be positive or negative, synonyms or random thoughts. Circle the words on the page that you've heard associated with not drinking. In the space below, jot down where this thought originated (if you can recall) and why it has that connotation. And no judgment here—we all see things differently. Also, you're the only one who's going to see these answers any-way. So, get as detailed—and candid—as you'd like.

_____

_____

_____

_____

_____

_____

_____

_____

_____

_____

_____

_____

_____

_____

PREGNANT
HEALTHY
RESPONSIBLE
HAPPY
SICK
BUTTONED UP
SMART
BORING
STRICT
LONELY
OUT OF CONTROL
UNTRUSTWORTHY
SERIOUS

Friends Who Drink Together ...

"DRINKING BUDDIES" IS A TERM that has entered the vernacular of fraternity brothers, business professionals, parents across the country, and people of every age, socioeconomic background, and friend group in between. The funny/interesting/remarkable thing about this term is that we all know what it means—the people we meet up with to have a bevvy or two. And perhaps that's all we do with them. Or maybe it's more than that. Maybe they're the people you grew up with, or the people that you work and network with. Or they're the friends you met at a bar one day who became your after-work hangout crew. Wherever and whoever, there's always a story (usually a few). Where, when, and with whom do you usually drink? How does your night start? How does it end? What do you feel throughout that experience? List your drinking buddies and describe your experiences with them in the spaces provided.

1. Who: _____
   Where: _____
   When: _____

2. Who: _____
   Where: _____
   When: _____

3. Who: _____
   Where: _____
   When: _____

4. Who: _____

   Where: _____

   When: _____

5. Who: _____

   Where: _____

   When: _____

6. Who: _____

   Where: _____

   When: _____

7. Who: _____

   Where: _____

   When: _____

8. Who: _____

   Where: _____

   When: _____

9. Who: _____

   Where: _____

   When: _____

10. Who: _____

    Where: _____

    When: _____

11. Who: _____

    Where: _____

    When: _____

Drawing Conclusions

BUILDING ON THE PREVIOUS EXERCISE, draw three images—one in each of the three corresponding frames shown here—that represent 1) where, when, and with whom you usually drink; 2) how the night starts; and 3) how it ends. Within each image, indicate emotions, feelings, and state of mind via word and thought bubbles, facial expressions, and captions, if you so choose. You can recall a specific story or generalize your experience with a detailed picture or a simple squiggle. And, here's the best part: Whether you're a future Monet or a stick-figure artist, you will not be judged by your doodles. Promise.

1

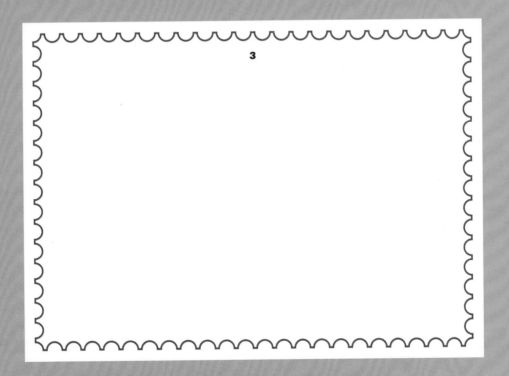

Charting Expectations

HERE'S THE CHART I DESPERATELY WISH I'd had leading up to my first dry challenge month (had I had the foresight to reflect on what was coming up). Using short, descriptive phrases, document your expectations or experiences with and without alcohol (the ups, the downs, and the weird, if applicable) in the following chart. Try to be as detailed as possible. Instead of "hard," try "challenging to relax." For now, just fill in the first two columns. You'll be coming back to this chart later in the book to fill in the third column. I got you started with a few suggestions for experiences to consider. Feel free to add more in the rest of the rows provided.

	WITHOUT ALCOHOL, NOW	WITH ALCOHOL, NOW	AFTER GOING DRY
My expectation(s) for my day:			
My experience(s):			
My nights are:			
My mornings are:			
My memories are:			

	WITHOUT ALCOHOL, NOW	WITH ALCOHOL, NOW	AFTER GOING DRY
My friends are:			

Preconceived Notions

NOW THAT WE'VE TOUCHED UPON your expectations and experiences abstaining from alcohol (not to mention personal feelings about drinking), let's dig into some outside beliefs. There are many common misconceptions about going dry that the population at large believes. In this exercise, we're going to make a list of these misconceptions and rephrase them to be more reflective of the truth. I've provided a few examples that I've heard many times (if you've had these thoughts yourself, no judgment here). Complete the exercise by writing down the misconceptions you've heard or had about going dry in the column on the left and then rephrase them to be supportive of your dry journey in the column on the right.

PHRASE	REPHRASE
"People who don't drink are boring."	People who don't drink are more present.
"Parties without alcohol are no fun."	People make the party—not the booze.

PHRASE	REPHRASE

Charting Your Cocktails

GRAPH YOUR GIN AND TONICS, MARGARITAS, martinis, glasses of wine, and other alcoholic beverages over the past week, as well as any nonalcoholic beverages you consumed while out and about (or in!). Nonalcoholic drinks include NA wines, beers, spirits, cocktails, sodas, sparkling waters, fruit juices—literally whatever! (If charts and graphs

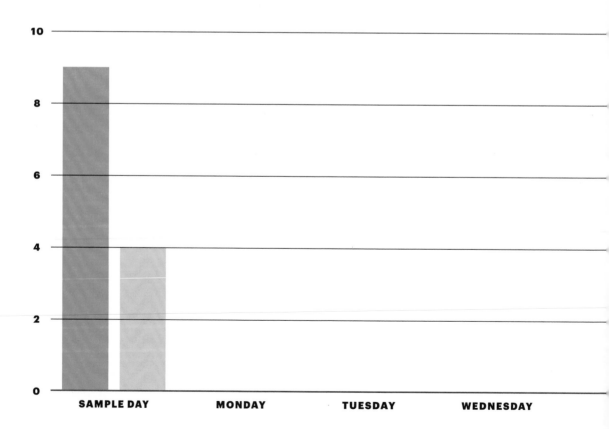

give you horrible flashbacks to eighth grade math class, don't worry. There's nothing very complicated here, and I've included a "sample day" in the following table for your reference). If you're having trouble remembering exactly what you had to drink (both boozy and otherwise), or you're a little fuzzy on the details (half a drink of this, a sip of that), you can refer to your receipts, phone a friend who was there, or simply take an educated guess. The closer to accurate you are, the better, but don't worry—it isn't 100 percent necessary to be 100 percent perfect. I promise no one is going to audit you later.

■ Alcoholic Beverage   ■ Nonalcoholic Beverage

| THURSDAY | FRIDAY | SATURDAY | SUNDAY |

Note to Self

HERE'S A POTENTIALLY SEMI-AWKWARD request . . . write a note to your drunk self. Do you wish you didn't text your ex? Or leave your credit card at the bar? Not shaming you (or anyone else), as we've all done things or forgot to do things while inebriated. I, for one, have returned home and didn't send the "I'm home safe!" text message to my friends, which sent some of them into a worrying tailspin because a) I swore I would, b) I had a great track record of doing so, and c) cities can be a not-so-safe place for tipsy individuals, especially after a certain hour (just listen to any true-crime podcast and/or read the headlines). For what it's worth, I thought I responded. Or maybe I started to but didn't hit send . . . Anyway, in this note, you can be as detailed as you'd like by referencing past events (i.e., that one time at your best friend's birthday) or just keep things short, sweet, and general. In the end, remember that it's important to reflect on these moments as opportunities to improve or change future situations and solidify any goals, new directions, or expectations you have for yourself. You might not feel great after completing this exercise (that's normal!) and perhaps you'll want to issue an apology to someone you wronged (which could be a good idea). The point is, we've all been there. And writing your wasted self a little note might help you express what you're looking to gain, achieve, and reflect upon in the coming weeks and months.

Once you're done, don't forget to sign and date it! Soberly, [yours truly].

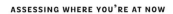

Goal Setting

ALL OF THE PREVIOUS ACTIVITIES have led us to the last exercise in this chapter: goal setting! You're going to be writing out your goals for the next month, three months, six months, a year; the time frame is up to you (though I recommend starting with at least a month). Write your goals in the blank spaces provided. Memorize them (or don't). Tear out this page and keep it in your back pants pocket (or leave it intact because you don't want to destroy your book, or library property!).

It's okay if your goals change over time. In January 2017, my goal was to finish the month without alcohol. And win a silly bet so I could enjoy a free meal courtesy of my friend (who lost our bet). By fall of 2023—nearly eight years later—my goal was to give up alcohol for three and a half months in order to properly train for and run the 2023 New York City Marathon. What a difference a couple of years makes, right? What started as a spontaneous challenge turned into a lifestyle that inspired bigger goals.

I've got to say, I don't recommend starting with a hefty goal like running 26.2 miles (on a whim) without consulting your physician, getting proper running shoes, and committing to months of training . . . but if that's in the cards for you, go for it. Or, start slow and complete one dry month. The choice is yours. And your goals are yours. Write them down here. You can categorize them by day, week, month, or year.

Also—for the record—you don't have to create bigger, elaborate goals week after week or year after year. Going dry for any amount of time is great enough as it is. No ifs, ands, or buts.

TIME	GOAL
(Sample) Month 1	Don't drink.
(Sample) Week 1	Order a mocktail in a bar instead of a cocktail.
(Sample) Week 2	Replace friend happy hour with a game night.

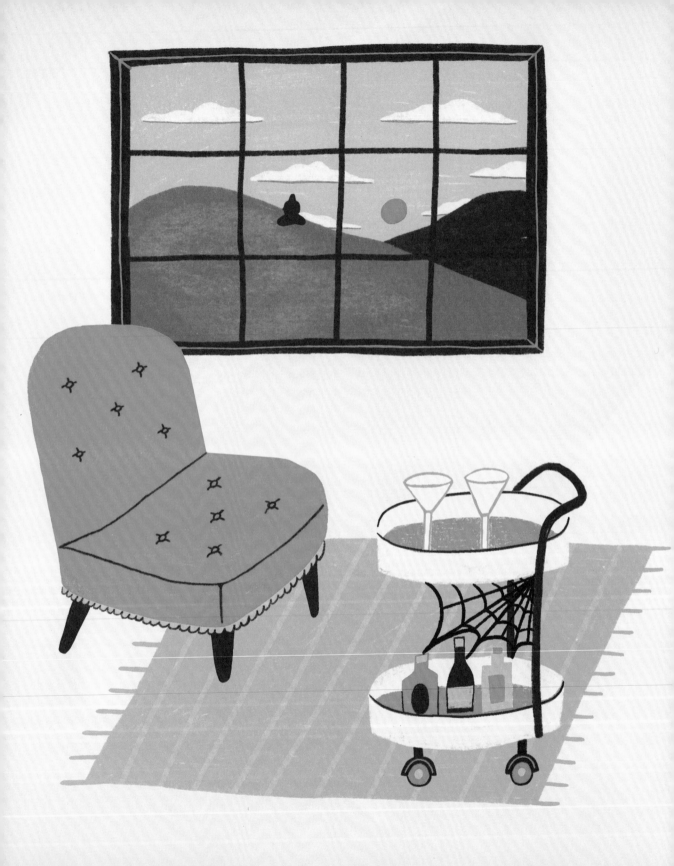

2

Discovering the Benefits of Living Alcohol-Free

ASK ANYONE—INCLUDING ME—what they noticed when they gave up alcohol, and they'll more than likely give you *something* positive to look forward to. It's true that going dry isn't all sunshine, but, as you very well know, drinking isn't either.

That being said, choosing to drink a nonalcoholic beverage instead of a full proof one, or deciding to participate in a non-alcohol focused activity versus imbibing at the bar, can bring about some surprising benefits, even beyond saving a few bucks, trying something new, and avoiding a killer hangover.

In my personal experience, I have nothing less than cherished (yes, cherished!) the uninterrupted sleep, lack of dizziness and dehydration, and the clearer skin I got from giving up alcohol. And those are just the physical benefits! As far as other perks go, I've saved hard-earned paychecks instead of spending them on expensive cocktails. I've made new friends over non-drinking activities (i.e., people who prefer skipping the drinks and waking up early and clearheaded). I've saved myself hours upon hours of late nights that turn into early mornings and instead used that energy to do things I love and find new hobbies (à la running long distances on the weekends—who knew!).

The *most enjoyed, best ever* benefits of going dry differ from person to person, based on their overall lifestyle and what means the most to them. If saving money is a priority, that might be your number one benefit for going dry. If you're someone who hates consuming empty calories—voilà! Abstaining from alcohol is a surefire way to help you do just that.

Anyway, enough rambling about rewards! Let's get to the good stuff—i.e., how to thrive on your dry journey, and what this looks like IRL, starting with that very first day . . .

Day One

HELLO THERE! CONGRATS ON MAKING IT to your first day of going dry.

As luck would have it, the first day of my first dry challenge *really* started with a challenge. I was at brunch in New York City on New Year's Day with five friends. The waiter brought over six complimentary tequila shots: one for each person at the table. (Yikes.) As I had just proposed my Dry Month bet—and agreed to the terms—about twelve hours prior, this unexpected gift of free tequila immediately became my now-or-never moment.

And I have to admit, as someone who did not prepare at all for a dry month, never mind a moment of serious temptation on day one, my reality was thrust right in front of me. Did I feel great about this whole going dry thing, at that very moment? No. Refusing complimentary tequila was certainly not a "benefit" I signed up for. The opposite actually.

The moral of the story is that on day one, you may not feel your absolute best. In fact, most of the benefits will come during later days.

Before you start to feel the perks, what are you feeling and how are you feeling about your first official dry day? Do you feel pressure? Excitement? Anxiety? Let it out. Are you hungover? Be honest. (No judgment here.) Did you put a bedsheet over your bar cart or prepare in any way? Whatever your vibe is today, write about it. This is your day one.

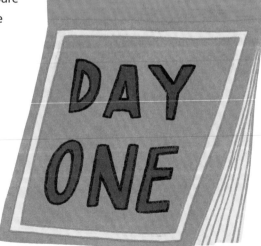

Circle Your Ideal Booze-Free Benefits

NOW THAT YOUR ADVENTURE in abstaining from alcohol is underway, what specific benefits are you hoping to gain from this experience? Circle the possible benefits from the following list. We're going to get into many of these in greater depth in the upcoming prompts, so for now, just think generally. And there are no wrong answers, so fill in anything that might be missing from the list.

More energy	Increased productivity	Other: _____
Elevated mood	Fewer mood swings	_____
Zero hangovers	Clearer skin	_____
Additional free time	Better sex	_____
More intentional dates	Improved digestion	_____
Better sleep	Healthier diet	_____
Focus	Financial savings	_____
Feeling accomplished	Fewer misunderstandings	_____

Rewriting a Very Bad Day

BAD DAYS AREN'T MADE BETTER with booze . . . they're made better with ice cream! Just kidding (well, actually . . .). All joking aside, alcohol often makes the bad days even worse by affecting not just your physical health but your mental health as well. After all, alcohol is a depressant. A clearer head and an elevated mood are major benefits of going dry. For this prompt, reach deep into your memory vault and recall a bad day that involved alcohol. Got it? Now, consider how this day could have gone had you been sober. Rewrite the memory as a dry day in the space provided. Better? I bet.

_____

_____

_____

_____

_____

_____

_____

_____

_____

_____

Sleepy Time, Part One

THIS IS ONE OF MY FAVORITE TOPICS when it comes to going dry. Let's get into the subject of shut-eye. Think about what your sleep is like when you've had a few drinks. What's your routine like? Do you feel super well rested? (I'm guessing not, especially after a round of drinks that ended at 3 a.m.) Note your experiences (hours slept, number of wake-ups, dreams, etc.) in the space provided. Feel free to use a sleep tracker, if you have one, to confirm this data or just go off memory.

Sleepy Time, Part Two

NOW THAT YOU'VE EXAMINED what your sleep patterns are like when you're drinking, in this exercise you're going to explore what your patterns are like when you go dry. But first, a story.

Before my first dry challenge, I thought I was a terrible sleeper due to work anxiety and my busy schedule at the time. I would wake up in the middle of the night (read: 3:30 a.m.). Sometimes I would fall back asleep. Sometimes I would just be up for the day. It's as unhealthy, tiresome, and downright sad as it sounds. As it turns out, my wakings weren't because I was stressed out (well, not all of them). The majority of them were caused by the alcoholic beverages I was drinking hours before. It was both infuriating and freeing to figure this out. Now it's your turn to see for yourself.

In this exercise, you're going to keep count of how many restful and uninterrupted nights of sleep you're able to rack up without booze. Again, if you have a sleep-tracking device available to you, use it! If not, your experiences will be more anecdotal and general, but still valuable! Leave a few blank rows at the end of this chart. Sweet dreams . . .

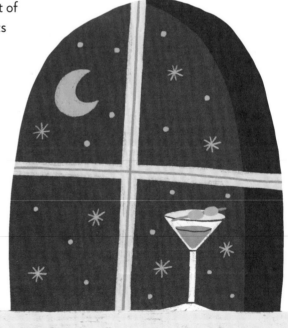

NIGHT	WOKE UP DURING THE NIGHT	DREAMS (GOOD/BAD)	HOW MUCH REM SLEEP (EST.)?	HOW MUCH DEEP SLEEP (EST.)?	EASY TO WAKE?	ADDITIONAL DETAILS
1	Woke up 3×	Bad dream about falling	1 hour	1 hour	Was up before my 7 a.m. alarm at 5 a.m.	Stressed about work. No hangover
2	Did not wake	Good dream about puppies	3 hours	4 hours	Got out of bed naturally, felt well-rested	No hangover

"Do You Want to Get a Drink Some Time?"

DATING AND ALCOHOL ARE COMMONLY assumed to go hand in hand, so if you're worried that going dry might have a dampening effect on your dating life, I don't blame you. But I'm going to challenge this assumption and argue that better dating is actually one of the best benefits of being booze-free.

The truth is, it's much easier to evaluate if someone is the right match without alcohol and its distractions. In fact, going dry can be an interesting test case for a potential match. When I was single and dating, it became clear very quickly that people who didn't respect my choice to go dry were probably not going to be my person. If they didn't like something I was (healthily!) pursuing for a month, I had to wonder if they'd respect my other goals and choices. Another benefit to dating without alcohol is getting to partake in activities that you love to do, and wouldn't be able to do if you had a bevvy in hand. (Boozy rock climbing, anyone? Yeah, no thanks.) We've all had dates like this in the past, and they're usually really pretty great, right? Doing the things you love that don't involve beer, wine, or cocktails means that you can show a potential partner more of your personality, interests, and who you really are.

What potential benefits have you experienced while going on dry dates? What positive outcomes can occur when you go on dates without alcohol?

Tally Up

FINANCIAL BENEFITS, IN THIS ECONOMY? I'll take it! Saving money is—undeniably—an excellent benefit of going dry. In this exercise, you're going to learn just how much all those drinks (and the extras that come with them) add up. Pull up your bank account, credit card statement, and/or your Venmo transactions from this month one year ago (or another month when you were still drinking). Add up all your boozy drink orders, handles of liquor, Ubers/taxis, hangover remedies, and any other foods and snacks that were a result of the late-night boozy munchies (you know the ones).

Calculate your grand total here: $_____ USD.

Does this total shock you? What could you have spent this money on, if not booze? Also take into consideration that a friend might have paid for your bevs here and there, your ride, or maybe spotted you $20 USD for a late-night snack on the way home. At the end of the day, someone (you or your bestie or your partner) is saving money when you don't drink, and that hard-earned cash could be put toward financial milestones or other things you're interested in experiencing, pursuing, or acquiring. Got any thoughts on what those could be? Note them here!

_____

_____

_____

_____

_____

_____

Crunch the Numbers

NOW THAT YOU HAVE ALL OF THAT spending data in front of you and you've done a little thinking about what you could spend that cash on instead, here's your opportunity to really crunch the numbers and set some goals to help you obtain the items or experiences you are pining after. Use the following chart to determine how many drinks you'd need to pass up to get to your goal purchase. In the first column, write down your goal purchase (concert tickets, new tattoo, trip to Hawaii, etc.) and the total cost of that purchase. In the second column, write down the number of drinks, multiplied by the rough cost of the drinks, that make up the equivalent amount. In the third column, consider how many drinks you have a week, and then calculate how many weeks it would take you to save up that amount if you simply gave them a pass. Fill this out for as many goals as you like!

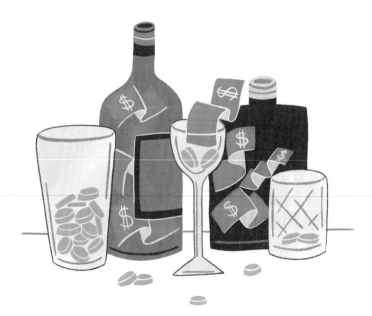

GOAL PURCHASE	# OF DRINKS AND COST OF DRINKS	WEEKS TO OBTAIN GOAL
Concert tickets: $400 USD	20 (drinks) × $20 USD	5 (if drinking 4 drinks each week)

Questioning Your History

NO MORE TIPSY EMBARRASSING MOMENTS: Yep, that's definitely a perk! Inebriated times can inspire the slow death of one's ego. Sometimes we brush off silly happenings, and sometimes they haunt us in our dreams and waking hours. I . . . am not going to share any personal regrets here, but you can privately! In the space provided, write about your most unfortunate experience from the past year—or ever—that occurred when alcohol was involved. Put pen to paper and spare no detail of the incident and the aftermath. It's only human to think, "How could that have gone differently?" We can't undo the past. But, it is possible to rewrite the story as if you were dry and explore how you would have handled the occurrence differently, if you hadn't been drinking. Would your whole life be different? (Maybe.) Would a friendship still be intact? (Perhaps.) Work through these questions as you reflect on a difficult moment in your history, and as you make room to explore different experiences in the future.

_____
_____
_____
_____
_____
_____
_____
_____
_____
_____
_____
_____
_____
_____
_____
_____
_____
_____
_____
_____
_____

So. Much. Time.

WHILE GOING DRY, YOU MIGHT FIND yourself bored—not boring!—as you suddenly recover all that time you used to spend working toward, or dealing with, a hangover. The funny thing about time is that we all agree we never have enough of it. We're bogged down with work or family responsibilities, on top of (trying) to take care of ourselves, eat right, and get enough sleep and exercise. And yet, we voluntarily lose so much time to drinking and its aftermath. Just how many canceled plans or days called off of work have you experienced due to hangovers and exhaustion? Of course, work is nonnegotiable for most of us; that time's on lock. But, outside of the (real or virtual) office, there are many hours in the day, especially during the weekends, to participate in fun, productive, new things. I realized I had more focus at work during my dry months, so my weekends were less about playing catch-up with my emails and more about taking small vacations out of town. I got to see more of the world, and the city in which I live, just by going dry.

Now it's your turn to think about how to fill the time you're getting back by going dry. Following is a weekly calendar you can use to fill your newfound free time with fun activities you love. For example, you could schedule workout classes, hikes, coffee shop visits, music lessons, concerts, theater performances, meditation, and travel. You could get involved with community service or sign up for local events by doing a little internet research about what's available and coming to town. Event websites usually have something for everyone. Now, go get planning!

SUN	MON	TUE	WED	THU	FRI	SAT

Photo Shoot

NOT TO SOUND SHALLOW, but this is a fact: Alcohol is terrible for your skin. Alcohol dehydrates the skin and can make wrinkles more visible and make acne and rosacea more prominent. While most of the beauty world is focused on serums, cleansers, and eye creams (totally valid, by the way), one of your best defenses is simply passing up the opportunity to drink. It's also a fact that after you've been drinking, you're less likely to remove your makeup (which clogs pores) and/or wash your face (and take out your contacts—eeeek!). So there's that, too!

Flip through photos from last month, last year, or any given week when you were drinking. Compare that photo to what your skin looks like today (take some pics), and again when you complete this workbook (snap some more photos). Do you notice a difference in texture? Brightness, dullness, or glow? How about inconsistencies, acne, or pore size? (If your skin is perfect throughout this entire exercise, well, then you won the lottery for best skin ever!) Write down any differences you notice here.

_____

_____

_____

_____

_____

_____

_____

_____

Health Check

WE TOUCHED UPON THE BENEFITS of more quality sleep and clearer skin, but some not-so-obvious internal health benefits include more energy, better digestion, and improved blood pressure. If you've recently visited your doctor for a checkup, you may have discussed some of these topics. If not, now is the perfect time to self-evaluate and research where your health stands (and what you're potentially looking to improve). When I'm going dry, I don't always feel "super," but on average, my self-rankings are typically higher on the scale than during nondry times in my life (especially in the energy-level category).

On a scale from 1 (awful) to 5 (super), rate how you feel now about the following subjects as they pertain to your body and self. When you finish this workbook, come back and rate the same elements. And if you want to try to predict the future, give it a shot (no pun intended) and write down what you think (or what you hope) will happen to your body in the coming days, weeks, and months while going dry.

ENERGY

5	4	3	2	1
Super	Good	Fair	Not Great	Awful

INFLAMMATION

5	4	3	2	1
Super	Good	Fair	Not Great	Awful

DIGESTION

5	4	3	2	1
Super	Good	Fair	Not Great	Awful

MENTAL HEALTH

5	4	3	2	1
Super	Good	Fair	Not Great	Awful

CLEARHEADEDNESS

5	4	3	2	1
Super	Good	Fair	Not Great	Awful

IMMUNE SYSTEM

5	4	3	2	1
Super	Good	Fair	Not Great	Awful

GENERAL FITNESS

5	4	3	2	1
Super	Good	Fair	Not Great	Awful

_____

_____

_____

_____

_____

_____

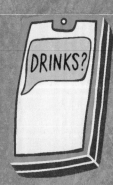

3

Roadblocks

THERE ARE MANY BENEFITS to going dry, but unfortunately, that doesn't mean the path is easy to navigate. There will be hurdles along the way, appearing in many forms—naysayers (including friends, family, and strangers), events on the calendar that are focused on alcohol or have an alcohol component, and other day-to-day incidents, irritants, and emotions that might tempt you to give up the whole thing.

As annoying as it sounds, these hindrances are all part of the ride. Yes, there will be roadblocks, but more important than anticipating these rocks in your path is knowing how to prepare for them.

Have friends getting married? Good for them! There will probably be a champagne toast—but not for you. That birthday on the calendar? Let's plan to hit the piñata rather than the piña coladas. Cool?

Even if you're not someone who plans your every single move, you'll quickly adapt to opting for other consumables (like cake!), and soon navigating these situations will become a piece of cake—or at least less of a roadblock and more of a swerve to the mocktail portion of the open bar.

In fact, during my first dry wedding, I did just that. I opted for a nonalcoholic beverage and all of the cake . . . which I highly recommend. Unless you are diabetic, gluten-free, or have another dietary restriction. Then do not listen to any advice I've given in the last paragraph.

Holidays are often a particular challenge—Thanksgiving, Christmas, New Year's, etc. But with a little preparation, you'll be ready to celebrate, give gifts, and socialize while staying dry. In these next few exercises, you'll discover how.

What Are You Up to These Days?

BY NOW, YOU MAY HAVE NOTICED a difference in how you're spending your time and with whom you're socializing. Or maybe not! Maybe you still go to bars and abstain from drinking while your colleagues and peers imbibe. To each their own! For me, as time went by, I started spending less time with some people I used to see often round the bar scene, because I was spending more time on relationships and activities in my life that weren't alcohol-centric.

When passing up alcohol, or activities centered around drinking, who do you see less of, and why? How do you feel about that? Do you find that you keep the same company outside of the bar scene, or are you still going to the same places and having just as much fun? Do you feel pressured by your environment or social group to drink? Note down your thoughts here.

_____

_____

_____

_____

_____

_____

_____

_____

_____

Welcome to the Mocktail Party

ONE OF THE BEST THINGS ABOUT going dry in the twenty-first century? The mocktails! While past nondrinkers were stuck with plain sparkling water or orange juice, today, bar and restaurant menus are overflowing (pun intended) with nonboozy bevs of all flavors, colors, and textures. This prompt is all about turning what seems to be an obstacle ("What do I drink instead?") into a fun exploration of the zero-proof world. In the space provided, research or brainstorm a list of five to six delicious nonalcoholic drinks to try during this time period. If you need a little inspiration to get started, here are three easy recipes (with common bar materials) that you can make at home or kindly ask the bartender to mix, muddle, shake, and stir so you can still have a drink in hand, even if it doesn't include the hard stuff.

1. _____

2. _____

3. _____

4. _____

5. _____

6. _____

Nogroni
(Nonalcoholic Negroni)

INGREDIENTS
1½ oz (44 ml) Free Spirits The Spirit of Milano or nonalcoholic aperitivo of choice
1½ oz (44 ml) Free Spirits The Spirit of Gin or nonalcoholic gin of choice
1½ oz (44 ml) Free Spirits The Spirit of Vermouth Rosso or nonalcoholic vermouth of choice
Orange peel, for garnish

METHOD
1 In a rocks glass, combine the spirits over one large ice cube and stir.

2 Garnish with an orange peel.

Faux Mule

INGREDIENTS
2 oz (59 ml) Fluère Spiced Cane or nonalcoholic rum of choice
4 oz (118 ml) ginger beer
½ oz (15 ml) lime juice
Lime wedge, for garnish

METHOD
1 Combine the spirits and lime juice in a glass over ice and stir.

2 Garnish with a lime wedge.

Mio Fresca

INGREDIENTS
5 strawberry halves, divided
1 oz (30 ml) lemon juice
1 oz (30 ml) agave syrup
3 oz (89 ml) Mionetto Alcohol-Removed Sparkling Wine or sparkling non-alcoholic white wine of choice
Lemon wheel, for garnish

METHOD
1 Muddle four strawberry halves in a cocktail shaker.

2 Add lemon juice and agave syrup.

3 Fill three-quarters of the shaker with ice.

4 Shake vigorously.

5 Strain into a white wine glass over ice.

6 Top with nonalcoholic sparkling wine and garnish with remaining strawberry half and lemon wheel.

Wedding Bells

WEDDINGS—IT'S LIKELY THAT if you're attending one (or planning one! Congrats, if so!), there might be a champagne toast and curated cocktails for the couple. If you are part of the bridal party or a groomsman, it's become tradition to sip alcoholic beverages as you get ready for the day ahead.

But weddings are supposed to be a celebration of the couple's love for one another, not the open bar (. . . right?). When you aren't drinking, you can be more clearheaded and present during a really special, important day—whether that day is focused on you or people you care about.

In an effort to be part of the party (and give life to the party, without an alcoholic beverage), here are some of my simple recommendations:

- **Eat cake:** Grab a slice of cake (or two). Help people acquire their slices of cake. Take pictures of the newlyweds as they smash cake into each other's faces.

- **Dance:** Hit the dance floor on your own, with someone in the wedding party, and definitely with the grandparents! Have them show you some moves. Teach them some, too.

- **Drink, in your own way:** Try a nonalcoholic drink when you get thirsty from all that disco dancing!

Now that you have some ideas on how to keep yourself busy (and happy) during a wedding, jot down other ways to keep yourself from boozing the night away.

- _____
  _____
  _____
- _____
  _____
  _____
- _____
  _____
  _____
- _____
  _____
  _____
- _____
  _____
  _____
- _____
  _____
  _____
- _____
  _____
  _____
- _____
  _____
  _____
- _____
  _____
  _____
- _____
  _____
  _____
- _____
  _____
  _____
- _____
  _____
  _____
- _____
  _____

Family Gatherings

WHETHER IT'S A HOLIDAY, a reunion, or another type of familial gathering, getting together can be stressful. The pressure of the holidays, paired with your mom's opinions and/or your dad's well-intentioned but aggressive questions, travel stress, and other uncontrollable elements, can be a lot.

While drinking is a common way to dissociate and relieve stress—instead try meditation or breath work.

I'm not a certified coach, but there's no denying breathing helps. Box breathing is one technique that's easy to remember. First off, take a deep breath by inhaling for four seconds. Hold the breath for four seconds, then exhale for four seconds. Repeat as needed until you feel calm. And especially don't forget to exhale (I always forget that part).

Now, there are a ton of step-by-step meditations and even more mantras on the internet that I could sprinkle in here for inspiration. My favorite one at the moment is, "This too shall pass." Because it's true. Time keeps ticking. The good and the bad are finite. And, because I don't know what exactly is stressing you right now, I can't pinpoint a more perfect quote that says, "You burned the turkey and that's okay," or "Why can't the airlines get everyone on the plane on time?" or "Aunt Gab just asked me if I'm dating anyone right now," in one quote as well as "This too shall pass." For a more specific mantra, try a search engine. I promise there are so many good quotes out there.

Try this breathing exercise and mantra the next time you're feeling the holiday stress and note how it worked/felt here.

Zero-Proof Gift Giving

THE HOLIDAYS SNEAK UP QUICKLY every year. In the months leading up to them, I always think of unique gifts to get friends and family, which I then completely forget when December comes around—ugh.

Holiday gift giving, host(ess) gifts, and even party favors often include alcohol (read: bottles of wine). And it's no surprise this is a go-to for many people who are gifting. The holidays usually include a ton of parties and celebrations, which also means a ton of—shock!—drinking. So a present of booze makes sense . . . but it's not optimal when you're going dry.

Instead, this year, try getting a little more creative than the standard bottle of red, white, rosé, or champagne for each of your loved ones. In the following chart, write out their name, an activity (or memory) you loved doing with them over the last year, and what an on-theme gift could be.

And, if you really can't figure out a present, nonalcoholic wine is a good look, too!

NAME	MEMORY	POSSIBLE PRESENT(S)
Hilary	Running, tennis, eating cake	Athletic shoes, a baking mixer
Leigh	Eating cookies	A cookie cutter, a bakery gift card

Ringing in the New Year

PERHAPS YOU'RE ALREADY NOT DRINKING in the days, weeks, and months leading up to January 1—amazing!

Drinking can be a big part of New Year's Eve plans for many, but it doesn't have to be the main event. Suggest a new activity that everyone can do, like karaoke, dancing, or anonymously writing down what you're looking forward to in the new year and having the host read it out loud. Or consider reviving some of the old-school traditions like eating grapes under the table for good luck.

Whether you're wearing sparkling accessories and dressing up, or collecting bets on who is going to leave the party before midnight, write down a few other ways to have fun during New Year's without a drink.

- _____
  _____
- _____
  _____
- _____
  _____
- _____
  _____
- _____
  _____

- _____
  _____
- _____
  _____
- _____
  _____
- _____
  _____
- _____
  _____
- _____
  _____
- _____
  _____
- _____
  _____
- _____
  _____
- _____
  _____
- _____
  _____

Romance Is in the Air, Alcohol Isn't

DATING AND ROMANCE. I DON'T BLAME YOU if you're a little nervous about this aspect of the dry life. But a little preparation can go a long way toward easing nerves. So, in this exercise, you're going to prepare for and then reflect on your dating experiences while dry by answering three questions:

1. **Plan how you are going to tell** your love interest that you aren't drinking right now.

2. **Note how you hope** it will be received.

3. **What will you say if** they are not accepting of your goals?

Or, if you already told your significant other that you aren't drinking:

1. **How did you tell them?** Spare no detail.

2. **How did the conversation go?** Walk us through it.

3. **How did you feel** while chatting about this? Was your beau respectful of your dry plans or combative? Curious, or interested, or something else entirely?

1 _____

_____

_____

_____

_____

_____

_____

_____

2 _____

_____

_____

_____

_____

_____

_____

_____

_____

3 _____

_____

_____

_____

_____

_____

_____

_____

Dry Dating Ideas

VALENTINE'S DAY IS A GREAT HOLIDAY FOR . . . marketing! But dating takes place year-round, so it's important to celebrate love (and the love of chocolate) during all 365 days of the calendar year.

In the space provided, list out activities you love to do by yourself, with friends or family, or dream of doing with a partner, and then add a romantic twist, sans alcohol. I've included some ideas to get you started.

ACTIVITY	ROMANTIC TWIST
Ice skating	With hot chocolate
Cooking classes	Making dishes for two, without cooking wine

ACTIVITY	ROMANTIC TWIST

The Birthday Conundrum

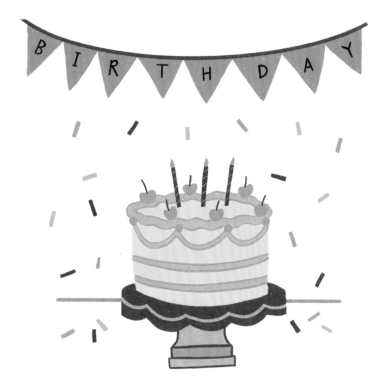

HAPPY BIRTHDAY! *Extends beverage glass and shouts "Cheers!" in unison.* Sounds familiar, right? This might have been the scene of every birthday you've had since your twenty-first (or even before!).

The last time I had a booze-free birthday was more recent than most—but when I think about not drinking on my birthday, it's another memory that comes to mind: the pool party I had when I turned nine. It was sunny, my friends were happily jumping into the water, and everyone wore brightly colored bathing suits. It was a great day all around. And I took a nap that afternoon.

Which poses the question: When was the last time you celebrated a birthday without alcohol? Was it as an adult? Even if the last one was during childhood, what was that experience like? How do you remember feeling that day? Could you recreate any (good) moments from that day and make your next birthday an alcohol-free event? Describe what that might be like.

_____

_____

_____

_____

_____

_____

_____

_____

_____

_____

_____

_____

_____

_____

_____

_____

_____

_____

_____

_____

Celebrating Milestones

IF YOU WERE HIRED FOR A NEW GIG, received a job promotion or a raise, or even just reached a new work or life milestone—congrats, you rockstar, you!

Instead of celebrating with booze (and whatever that might cost), let's brainstorm some other ways you can celebrate while staying dry. My favorite thing to do when I've met a goal is to dedicate "me" time during a weeknight or a weekend. It means I'm going to take a long walk, maybe window-shop or grab a small treat from the bakery. Sure, I can do this anytime, but it's a dedicated action that helps me honor whatever milestone I've accomplished.

List your ideas for booze-free milestone celebrations here!

- _____
  _____
- _____
  _____
- _____
  _____
- _____
  _____
- _____
  _____
- _____
  _____

- _____
  _____
- _____
  _____
- _____
  _____
- _____
  _____
- _____
  _____
- _____
  _____
- _____
  _____
- _____
  _____
- _____
  _____
- _____
  _____
- _____
  _____
- _____
  _____
- _____
  _____

Journal This, Journal That

IT GOES WITHOUT SAYING that at some point in your life, you're going to experience challenging feelings: sadness, grief, shame, awkwardness, negativity, and more—you get the gist. These feelings are a part of life and they test us. Instead of drinking away your feelings or bottling them up—an action that often makes the feelings worse—try sitting with and honoring the challenging feelings instead.

Journaling is a recognized technique for processing difficult emotions. Writing down day-to-day happenings, the good and not-so-great, can be meditative and help you reflect, learn more about yourself (and the world), inspire feelings of gratitude (for people, places, things, and circumstances), and more. So, go for it—detail the ups, the downs, the good, the bad, and the weird stuff that you come across, whether it involves booze or not. You can write about feelings that might make you feel like you want to drink away pain or discomfort. It's up to you. This is a safe space for sharing your feelings—even the ugly ones.

_____

_____

_____

_____

_____

_____

_____

_____

_____

Body Scan

STRESS AND ANXIETY ARE NO FUN for anyone, but drinking can actually make it worse (even if you think you're feeling calmer at first). The next time you're stressed, instead of drinking, try a body scan to help you return to the present, relax your body, and find calm.

First, find a place and position that's comfortable. (I recommend laying down.) Now begin mentally scanning your body, one part at a time, starting at the tips of your toes and moving up all the way to the crown of your head. Pay attention to how each body part feels as you visit it. Note where you're holding tension or stress. Write down where your body feels uncomfortable or at ease. Do this weekly or whenever you feel particularly stressed, and feel how your body changes over time without the presence of alcohol in your system. Describe your experiences in the space provided.

Practicing Booze Boundaries

PEER PRESSURE ISN'T FUN, and as many times as you explain yourself and politely refuse a drink, sometimes people don't get it. That's okay—you can't control everything, and sometimes people are just . . . people.

Here's something to practice the next time someone crosses a boundary, tries to pressure you into doing something you don't want to do, or just says something insensitive. Turn on your heels and walk away. That's it! It's time to go.

Okay—I admit, that sounds great in theory. But in reality, walking away might not be so easy. If you're stuck in a situation or conversation about going dry that you'd really rather not be in, it can be helpful to have a few stock phrases prepared to help you stay strong, hold your boundaries, and end the conversation as quickly and politely as possible. For example:

- **"Drinking is not in the plans for me tonight.** I have an early morning and don't want to sleep through my alarm. Have you ever done that?"

- **"Thanks for offering me a drink,** but I'm drinking [insert nonalcoholic beverage here] and have my hands full right now."

Now it's your turn. Following are a few examples of annoying, insensitive, or prying questions and comments you might get when people notice you're not drinking. In the space below each one, brainstorm and write down a firm response that you would feel comfortable giving in the moment. Then practice these until you feel ready to use them in real life.

Do you have a drinking problem? _____

_____

_____

Are you pregnant? _____

_____

_____

Isn't that kind of boring? _____

_____

_____

Why are you being such a buzzkill? _____

_____

_____

Are you just jumping on the dry bandwagon? _____

_____

_____

What's the point of a dry month if you're going to drink again,

anyway? _____

_____

_____

_____

JANUARY

SUN	MON	TUE	WED	THU	FRI	SAT
		1	WORK OUT	3	4	HIKE!
ME DAY ☺	7	8	9	10	AFTER WORK HAPPY HOUR	12
13	SOBER PAINT & SIP	15	CALL MOM	17	18	JEN'S WEDDING
20	21	22	HAWAII ←	☀	⌇	HAWAII →
27	28	29	30	PROJECT DUE		

4

Making It Fun
(Because It Is)

CHAPTER **3** WAS ALL ABOUT the hard parts of going dry; the challenges and obstacles you face when you give up alcohol. In this chapter, we're switching gears to talk about the fun side of things. Because it *is* fun—if you have the right mindset.

What are things that you enjoy doing in your time away from work and other responsibilities—without booze? Perhaps you think about spending time with your favorite people, laughing, joking, and bonding over shared experiences. Maybe your idea of fun is traveling, working on projects with your hands, reading, or showcasing your creativity through art.

However you define "fun," now is the time to lean into it. You can visit old pastimes and reignite your love of old hobbies. You can try new things and explore new places. In this chapter, we're going to be brainstorming all the ways you can bring booze-free fun back into your life. As you envision activities that make you smile, or dream up new ones, take note of the ideas that sound joyful—then do them.

When you take the reins and decide to lean into making plans that revolve around friends, building community, and doing the things you love, like traveling, going to events, or whatever makes you feel good, you're going to be a happier version of you.

Space for Change

BEFORE WE GET INTO THE BRAINSTORMING part of this chapter, let's consider how and where we've been using alcohol to bring the "fun factor" into our lives. Alcohol is often used to bring fun into less-than-fun spaces and situations (why else would work parties include so much booze?). But over time, it can start to take up a lot of space in your life, popping up in your work life, leisure time, relationships, etc.

Where in your life have you used alcohol to have fun? And what could you have done instead?

- _____
  _____
- _____
  _____
- _____
  _____
- _____
  _____
- _____
  _____
- _____
  _____

- _____
  _____
- _____
  _____
- _____
  _____
- _____
  _____
- _____
  _____
- _____
  _____
- _____
  _____
- _____
  _____
- _____
  _____
- _____
  _____
- _____
  _____
- _____
  _____

Find Your Friends

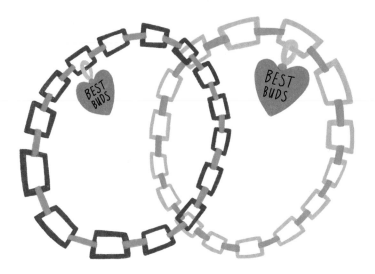

IN GRADE SCHOOL, THERE WERE so many opportunities to make friends. As an adult? Not so much. Making a new friend when you're a grown-up takes time and scheduling and a lot more effort—and luck. While making genuine connections is the goal, finding like-minded people can be as easy as a quick Google search, looking up events in your area that you enjoy attending, going to workouts or pop-ups that interest you, and/or joining a club—none of which will involve alcohol. In this exercise, think about things you like to do and places you like to hang out. Start with the following categories and expand to more specific interests. This will give you a nice list of ideas and places to start when you're ready to begin putting yourself out there (as a friend).

And it's important to remember that, unless you're headed to dry-specific events, you'll probably meet people who aren't sober-curious. With that said, you'll still want to be intentional about where you go and what activities you'll enjoy (without booze).

Activities I enjoy: _____

_____

_____

_____

_____

_____

Workouts/sports that interest me: _____

_____

_____

_____

_____

_____

Events I enjoy: _____

_____

_____

_____

_____

_____

Places I like to hang out: _____

_____

_____

_____

_____

_____

Itinerary Mock-Up

ONCE YOU'VE DONE YOUR RESEARCH and have a list of activities, events, and places to work with, it's time to do some planning. In this exercise, pick something from the list you made in the previous prompt and get ready to make new friends (or take old ones) on a nonalcoholic adventure. Here's how to plan a day (or night) out without booze. First, come up with an activity and a destination. Next, set a date and time. Once the logistics are set, mark your calendar and go!

Sounds easy, right? Well, if you're more of a planner, here are a few blank itineraries you can fill out when making your own plans.

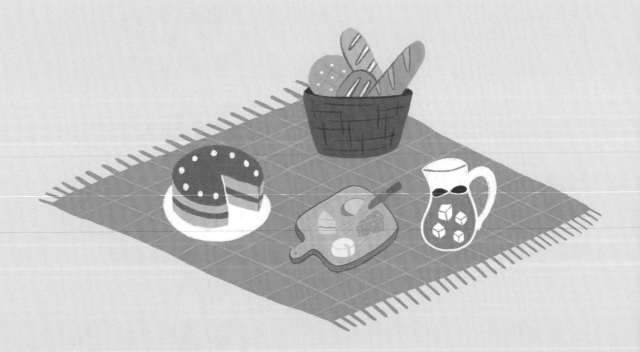

Activity: _____

Date: _____

Time/span of activity: _____

Location: _____

Invitees: _____

Rough costs: _____

What to bring for guests: _____

What guests should bring: _____

Food/beverage available: _____

Dress requirements: _____

Transportation requirements: _____

Notes: _____

_____

Activity: _____

Date: _____

Time/span of activity: _____

Location: _____

Invitees: _____

Rough costs: _____

What to bring for guests: _____

What guests should bring: _____

Food/beverage available: _____

Dress requirements: _____

Transportation requirements: _____

Notes: _____

_____

Mocktail Mixology

TIME FOR A LITTLE KITCHEN EXPERIMENTATION! You don't have to be a professional bartender to make a drink. While there are a ton of well-balanced, complex, and tasty mocktail recipes these days, sometimes you just want to hold a simple drink and call it your own. My go-to these days is sparkling water with a splash of pineapple juice, for what it's worth.

In this exercise, you're going to try your hand at a bit of home kitchen mocktail mixology. A lot of mocktails commonly start with some kind of nonalcoholic substitute for booze (wine, cider, beer, etc.), which is combined with a mixer or mixers and then garnished with some kind of botanical or fruit. Using the following lists of categorized ingredients, mix and match your nonalcoholic booze, mixers, and garnishes (or just mixers and garnishes if you prefer), add ice, and stir to discover something new! Write down your best (and worst) results. (Bonus: You could also invite friends over and make this a mocktail party. Just saying!)

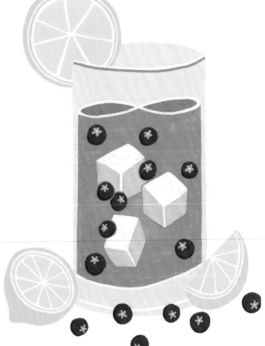

NA SPIRIT	COMMON MIXERS	GARNISHES
Nonalcoholic wine	Lemon juice	Lemon peel
Nonalcoholic beer	Lime juice	Salt (for rim)
Nonalcoholic cider	Orange juice	Sugar (for rim)
Nonalcoholic spirit	Ginger ale	Mint
	Tea	Rosemary
	Sparkling water	Candied ginger
	Pineapple juice	Orange peel
	Cranberry juice	Olives
		Berries
		Cherries

Name That Negroni . . .

WHILE WE'RE ON THE SUBJECT of making your own drinks—every great drink needs a fun name! In this exercise, we're going to be naming the recipes you developed in the previous prompt. If you're a creative person, give it your best shot (pun intended), but if naming a NA cocktail sounds stressful, don't fret—it doesn't have to be a crazy ordeal. In fact, I came up with a list of words that can help you name your drinks. Simply take two of the provided words (one from column 1 and one from column 2) and combine them! Or, use the word that corresponds to the first letter of your first name (column 1), and first letter of your last name (column 2) and let a higher power assign your drink a name.

MOCKTAIL NAMES

- _____
- _____
- _____
- _____
- _____
- _____
- _____
- _____
- _____
- _____
- _____

Column 1	Column 2
The	Dog
Nobody's	Favorite
First Place	Monster
Anybody's	Death
Green	Freeze
Purple	Revenge
Magnificent	Smoke
Slow	Surprise
Small	Cup
Sleepy	Dream
Stunning	Spoon
California	Chance
Major	Reward
Red	Honor
Ready	Gold
Sweet	Ticket
Adored	Danger
Crazy	Landing
Big	Bev
Early	Worm
Late	Breakfast
Cold	Night
Forever	Choice
Yesterday's	Joy
Future	Prize
Promised	Dust

Cheers to Not Drinking

YOU'VE GOT THE RECIPES. You've named them. What's left? The special glassware, of course! Even if you're not drinking, no one should miss out on the fun of sipping fancy drinks out of fun glassware—especially if you're drinking nonalcoholic varietals. You can, and should, get creative with it. After all, you're an adult. You can drink nonalcoholic sparkling wine out of a paper cup if your heart desires. (Cheers to that.) Choose the perfect vessels from the following selection of glassware to pour your mocktail creations into. You can label them by name, or color them in if you're feeling extra creative.

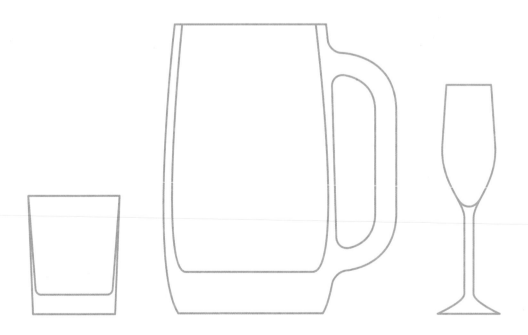

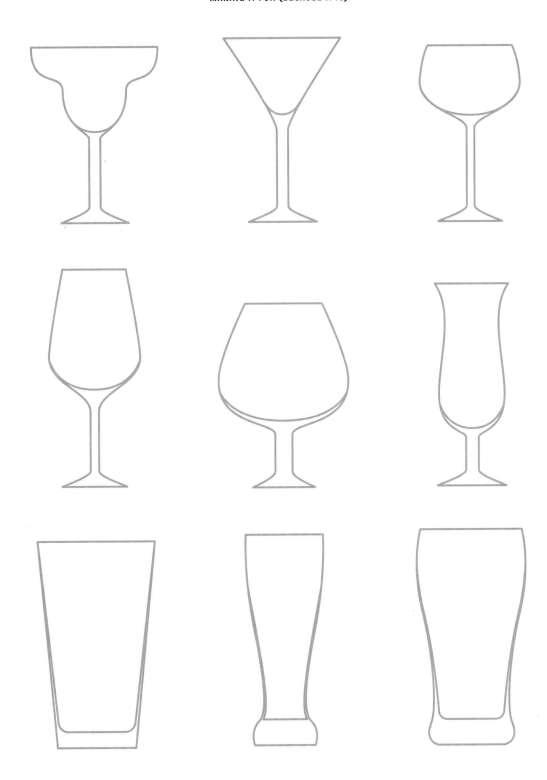

Cruise without Booze

IT'S TIME TO GET OUT OF TOWN! If you have the means and time to take a trip, vacation, or embark on a new adventure right now, this is absolutely the time to do it. Tons of hotels, resorts, and even airlines have nonalcoholic options these days. There are also retreats (and even certain countries) that do not serve alcohol. Where are your bucket list destinations? Write them down here, and what kind of stuff you want to do when you get there (that doesn't involve imbibing, obviously!).

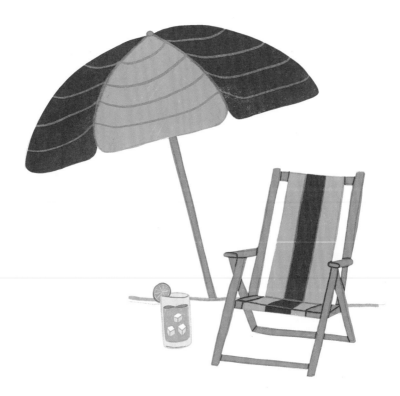

DESTINATION	ROMANTIC TWIST
Maui, Hawaii	Surf, swim

Where Not to Go

WHILE YOU'VE DEVELOPED SOME great ideas for where to go and what to do while you're going dry, the truth is that some places and activities are just not going to be fun right now. In fact, there are some places you may just need to avoid for the time being. Whether it's the atmosphere, memories of past events, or people that frequent certain places, all of these factors can contribute to making your dry goals difficult to achieve (read: not fun). Are there restaurants, bars, and venues that you frequent where you would feel pressured to drink? List them in the space provided. And, if you find yourself thinking about how it might be hard to say no, avoid these places or develop a plan (see "Practicing Booze Boundaries" on page 90).

- _____
  _____
- _____
  _____
- _____
  _____
- _____
  _____
- _____
  _____

-
-
-
-
-
-
-
-
-
-
-
-

Text Me!

YOU KNOW WHAT MAKES ANY EXPERIENCE more fun, or at least easier (usually)? Doing it with a friend. If you're lucky enough to have a friend who is going dry with you, then great! Your support person is built in. If not, pick at least one person in your life who supports your endeavors and ask them to be your "Sober Support Squad" so you can call or text them for help if you get stuck. It might not always come at a convenient time of day—and reaching out might not be necessary or happen at all—but in case you need to vent, curse (!), chat, or brainstorm with a trusted source about anything related to drinking, it's good to know that you have someone who will cheer you on to dry success. Make a list of personal contacts you can rely on in the space provided, and if you haven't already, reach out to them now so they can be ready to support you if and when the time comes.

Name: _____

Phone number: _____

Name: _____

Phone number: _____

Name: _____

Phone number: _____

Name: _____

Phone number: _____

Name: _____

Phone number: _____

Name: _____

Phone number: _____

Name: _____

Phone number: _____

Name: _____

Phone number: _____

Name: _____

Phone number: _____

Name: _____

Phone number: _____

Name: _____

Phone number: _____

Name: _____

Phone number: _____

Name: _____

Phone number: _____

Don't Text Me . . .

OKAY, SO, I DIDN'T WANT TO GO THERE . . . but it's the truth. Just like the places you're avoiding, there are people you might want to avoid, too. (Ugh, sorry—I had to say it!) It might not be forever, just for a little while, because if there's one thing that doesn't make any experience fun, it's doubters, naysayers, and Negative Nellies. In the space provided, make a list of not-so-supportive people that you might want to circle back with when you're feeling confident and unbothered by their views.

Name: _____

Phone number: _____

Name: _____

Phone number: _____

Name: _____

Phone number: _____

Name: _____

Phone number: _____

Name: _____

Phone number: _____

Name: _____

Phone number: _____

Name: _____

Phone number: _____

Name: _____

Phone number: _____

Name: _____

Phone number: _____

Name: _____

Phone number: _____

Name: _____

Phone number: _____

Name: _____

Phone number: _____

Name: _____

Phone number: _____

Resources for You

NO MATTER WHERE YOU ARE or what time of year it is, the thing about going dry is that you aren't alone. So many people have been in similar places, experiencing similar challenges, and, thanks to technology, it's easier than ever to find and connect with them. For this prompt, research and make a list of supportive books, media, podcasts, influencers, and authorities you can follow and refer to for tips, advice, and encouragement during this time. If you fill your feed with positive influences and fun inspiration, I guarantee you'll have a much better time!

- _____
  _____
- _____
  _____
- _____
  _____
- _____
  _____
- _____
  _____
- _____
  _____

- _____
  _____
- _____
  _____
  _____
- _____
  _____
- _____
  _____
- _____
  _____
  _____
- _____
  _____
- _____
  _____
  _____
- _____
  _____
  _____
- _____
  _____
  _____
- _____
  _____
  _____
- _____
  _____
  _____
- _____
  _____

Celebrate Dry Times!

QUICK QUESTION: Have you celebrated yourself lately? I mean, giving up booze is hard—alcohol is everywhere—but, no matter where you're at, I know you're doing your best. Let's celebrate that!

What does a dry celebration look like to you right now? Whether you're going out and drinking mocktails, having friends over for a dance party in your living room, buying a matcha latte, or chillin' by yourself and having an at-home spa day, congratulate and reward yourself accordingly! In the space provided, write down some ideas for how you want to honor your progress so far.

- _____
  _____
- _____
  _____
- _____
  _____
- _____
  _____
- _____
  _____
- _____
  _____

- _____
  _____

- _____
  _____

- _____
  _____

- _____
  _____

- _____
  _____

- _____
  _____

- _____
  _____

- _____
  _____

- _____
  _____

- _____
  _____

- _____
  _____

- _____
  _____

- _____
  _____

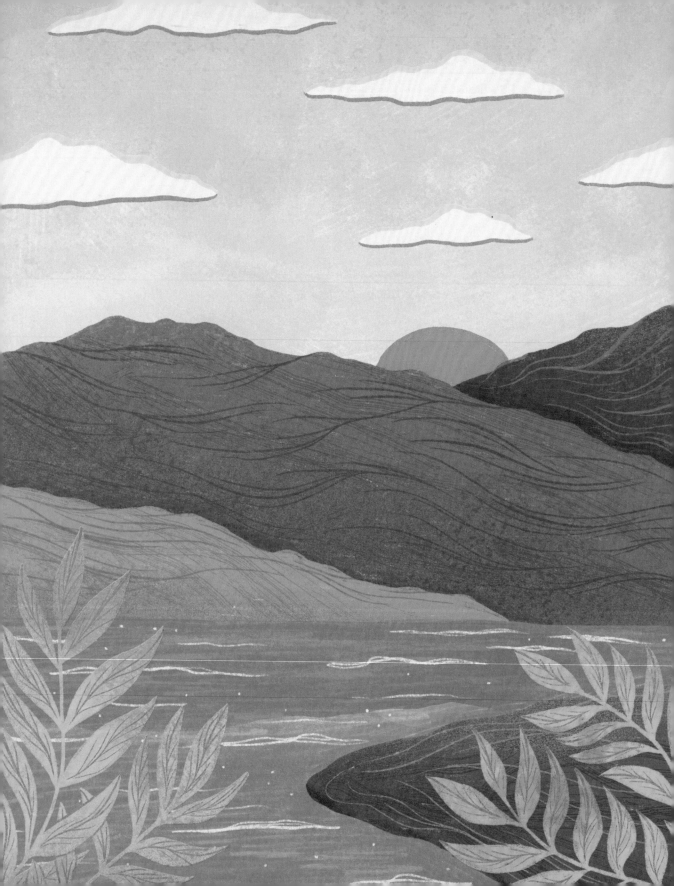

5

The Differences
So Far

ANY NEW PROJECT OR ROUTINE usually results in two kinds of changes: the ones you notice immediately and the ones that develop over time. When it comes to not consuming alcohol, it only takes one really good dry night out to see that you can have the same fun at a less expensive price point and without a hangover. At the same time, it might take a week or longer for your sleep to adjust to the point where you're catching regular undisrupted Zs. It will likely take even longer before you see other substantial differences, like weight loss, or notice major lifestyle changes.

All of that said, every positive change is welcome here! And in this chapter, you'll be counting them up and celebrating them. In my opinion, the best changes are the ones that you can't quite put your finger on, but you know they are taking place (like having a more upbeat attitude when alcohol isn't being consumed regularly). If you don't take the time to deliberately notice all the good stuff, it may pass you by. But not on my watch!

In the following prompts, we'll be looking back on chapter 2 a lot to compare your expectations with your reality. Have you experienced everything you thought you would? Let's find out.

Life Changes

NOW THAT YOU'VE EXPERIENCED dry life (or a snippet of it), what has changed in your life since the start of your dry journey? What has stayed the same? We're going to drill down further on this in the upcoming prompts, so for now, think big-picture stuff. What benefits do you clearly see/feel? Write down your answers to these questions in the space provided.

_____

_____

_____

_____

_____

_____

_____

_____

_____

_____

_____

_____

_____

_____

Throwback

FLIP BACK TO "CHARTING EXPECTATIONS" on page 28. In the chart there, you made notes on the expectations you had about experiencing life both with and without alcohol. Now it's time to fill in the third column, "After Going Dry," to reflect on what differences have taken place. After a month without booze, do you see an even bigger variance in your expectations for your life? Was this what you imagined would happen and what you'd be writing in the "after" column?

As you compare your notes, in the space provided, reflect on what differences are the most stark. How do they make you feel—proud, surprised, inspired to do more? Spare no detail!

_____

_____

_____

_____

_____

_____

_____

_____

_____

_____

I Love Love

FOR SOME, DRINKING CAN enhance social opportunities. For others, quite the opposite. Which begs the questions: How have your relationships—with friends/family/a partner or date—changed since going dry (if at all)? How have your social activities altered (if at all)? Chronicle a story in the space provided about how your relationship with a person close to you has shifted.

_____

_____

_____

_____

_____

_____

_____

_____

_____

_____

_____

_____

_____

Can I Ask You a Question?

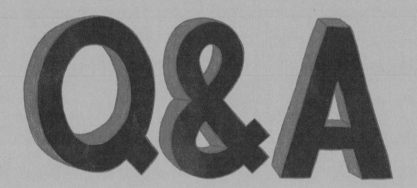

YOU'VE PROBABLY GOTTEN A LOT of interesting queries about this whole going dry thing over the last few weeks—some more personal than others. In the space provided, document what questions you received the most. How did each make you feel? How did you respond? What questions did you not like being asked and what did you like discussing?

_____

_____

_____

_____

_____

_____

_____

Ask Me Anything

ON THE OTHER HAND, maybe there were some details (big, small, fleeting, or permanent) you wanted to talk about but didn't have the opportunity to bring up. What do you wish people asked? What do you wish more people knew about not drinking (for any amount of time)?

_____

_____

_____

_____

_____

_____

_____

_____

_____

_____

_____

_____

Big Events

WEDDINGS. HOLIDAYS. MILESTONE MOMENTS. They all (usually) have drinks, and sometimes even an open bar . . . which is not conducive to helping attendees stay dry. Looking back, which big life event, holiday, celebration, or activity was the easiest or most accommodating when it came to not drinking? How about the least? What were you feeling during each experience?

_____

_____

_____

_____

_____

_____

_____

Show Me the Money, Honey!

FLIP BACK TO "TALLY UP" (page 52). How has your relationship with alcohol changed as it relates to money? Review what you used to spend on alcohol. How does it compare to recent weeks? Are you spending your hard-earned cash on something different these days?

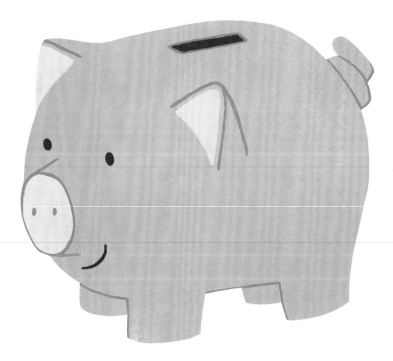

More Dates, Fewer Drinks

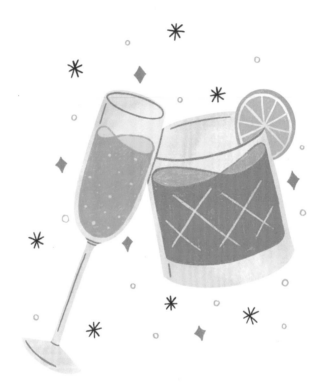

BACK ON THE NOTE OF DATING (or your relationship with your partner): Since we brought up sober dating, how did not drinking affect your relationship/spending time together? Describe your best date or romantic experience without alcohol in the last few weeks.

More Zs

WHETHER YOU USE A SLEEP-TRACKING device, smart bed, or nothing at all—how has your shut-eye quality changed each night? Flip back to "Sleepy Time, Part Two" (page 48) to fill in the blank rows and see if your sleep has improved since you last had a sip of alcohol. Reflect on your findings below.

_____

_____

_____

_____

_____

_____

_____

_____

_____

_____

_____

_____

_____

_____

_____

_____

_____

Cutting Booze and Cutting Calories

WHETHER YOU HAVE WELLNESS GOALS that include weight loss or not, alcohol does affect how digestion takes place and the food choices we make. On that note, what are some of your go-to drinking snacks (when you are in dire need of munchies) and your favorite hangover foods? This can be anything from pizza to fast food chicken nuggets, to greasy BLTs and bacon, egg, and cheeses in bed. (No judgment.) Now that I've got you thinking of guilty pleasures: How often do you/have you ordered these items since not drinking? And how do you feel now? Are you making the same choices at the same time of night or day? Write about it in the space provided.

Managing Emotions

WHEN ALCOHOL IS INVOLVED, sometimes emotions can get intense. Now that you've been cruising along without booze, how are you feeling emotionally? Has the way you regulate your emotions changed? Do you express your emotions differently now?

_____
_____
_____
_____
_____
_____
_____
_____
_____
_____
_____
_____
_____

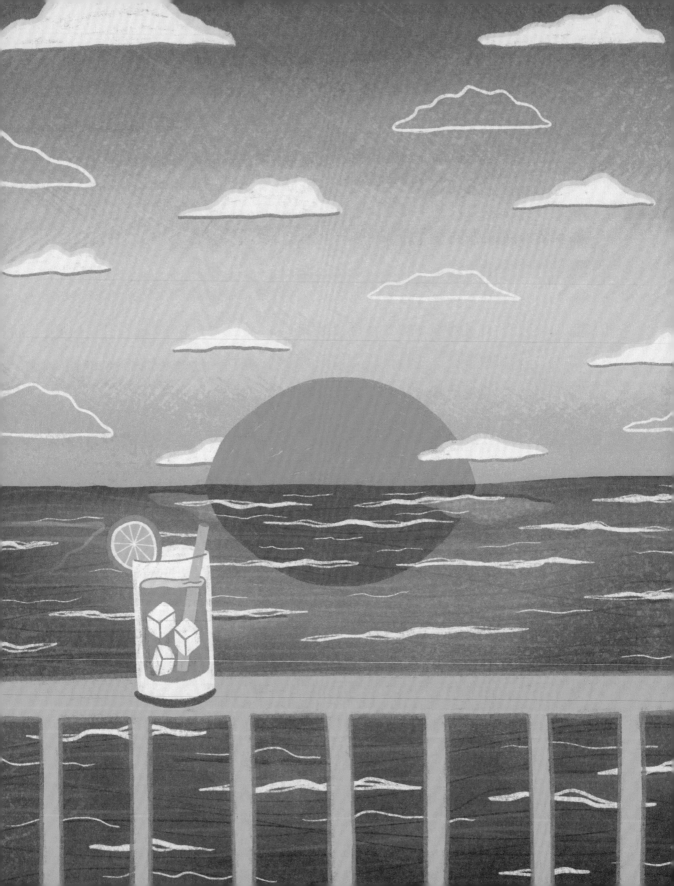

6

Sustaining New Lifestyle Habits

WHEN I STARTED DOING DRY MONTHS in 2017, I didn't know if I'd do another dry stint a year later. I certainly didn't expect to drink less in the long run. But both of those things happened. And all these years later, I participate in multiple dry months annually. (It was a surprise to me, too, but I digress . . .)

One of the great things about sustaining new habits is that you've already done the hard work of getting there, adapting, and making changes. Now all you have to do is continue on the path you've committed to (of course, with adjustment as needed) using the patterns you've created for yourself.

In this chapter, we'll review unique ways to sustain all of the good feelings, milestones, and memories that have resulted from your commitment to going dry, and sticking to it. It's also a time to reflect on where you are today and where you began. Alcohol is everywhere in our culture, and it's not an easy thing to give up, even for short periods of time. That said, I applaud you for any effort you've made up to this point and encourage you to keep going.

Carry This with You

YOU'VE SEEN CHANGES, experienced tough conversations and unwavering support, tried new things, and made new friends. So now the big question: What have you learned from all this? What lessons can you take from this experience into the next week, month, year, and beyond?

_____

_____

_____

_____

_____

_____

_____

_____

_____

_____

_____

_____

_____

_____

_____

_____

Keep the Good, Discard the Bad

WHETHER IT WAS ALL GOOD or more of a mix, chances are there's been a lot of new stuff going on in your life since you went dry. Write down the habits, relationships, and experiences you've developed over this journey that you want to keep going strong—whether that's attending nonalcoholic parties (or throwing your own) or sleeping better. The more details, the better! (*Psst.* You can also make a list of the things you tried that didn't work for you and you have no interest in revisiting . . . if you want!)

_____

_____

_____

_____

_____

_____

_____

_____

_____

Bar Cart Makeover

HERE'S A FUNNY THOUGHT: What is your bar cart doing right now? Or, if you don't have a cart, that space in your kitchen where you store the booze. If you're not drinking, what could you use this space for instead? Flowers? Art? Equipment storage for a fabulous new hobby? Write down some ideas here:

- _____

- _____

- _____

- _____

- _____

- _____

- _____

- _____
  _____
- _____
  _____
- _____
  _____
- _____
  _____
- _____
  _____
- _____
  _____
- _____
  _____
- _____
  _____
- _____
  _____
- _____
  _____
- _____
  _____
- _____
  _____

Stay Hydrated!

DIET SODA AT THE BAR is so last year. Just kidding—we still drink it. During your dry journey, you probably picked up a few new canned, bottled, steeped, and mixed drinks. What have been your favorites? Have you been enjoying nonalcoholic beverages and recipes or just been drinking more water? Hydration is important, so keep a record of where you go to get your favorite NA sips.

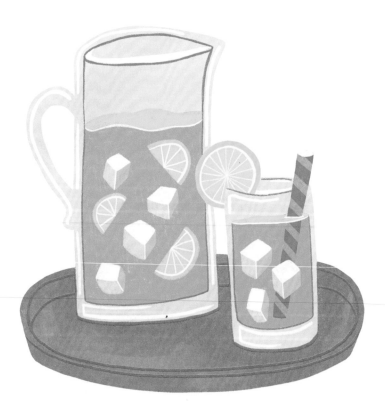

PLACE	ORDER	WHAT'S IN IT	PRICE	WHY DO YOU LOVE IT

New Goals

SORRY IF I DIDN'T WARN YOU EARLIER, but the reality is that when you stop drinking—or drink less—you might start making new goals for yourself. I certainly did. Don't be surprised if you find yourself making big plans when alcohol is not in the picture.

What goals or plans have you been inspired to pursue since going dry? These can be related to your health, spirituality, finances, social life, or something else entirely. Make a list and add deadlines for each specific feat to help you stay on track.

- _____
  _____
- _____
  _____
- _____
  _____
- _____
  _____
- _____
  _____
- _____
  _____
- _____
  _____

- _____
  _____
- _____
  _____
- _____
  _____
- _____
  _____
  _____
- _____
  _____
- _____
  _____
- _____
  _____
- _____
  _____
- _____
  _____
  _____
- _____
  _____
- _____
  _____
- _____
  _____
  _____

Advice Booth

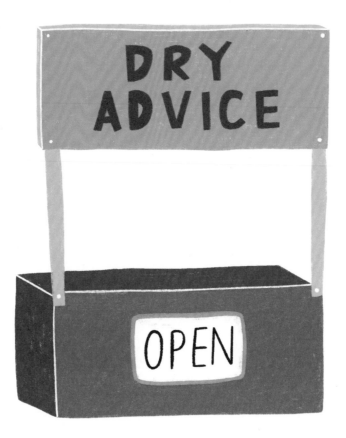

NOW THAT YOU'RE A GOING DRY VETERAN, you'll probably start getting questions from other sober-curious folks in your larger community. What are your best tips, suggestions, and advice for first-timers and/or future participants in a dry challenge? This can be anything from helpful hacks to deep thoughts you might have had about the experience.

Your Future Relationship

HAVING EXPERIENCED THE CHANGES, benefits, and challenges that come with going dry, what do you think your future relationship with alcohol will look like? If you had to define your new relationship with alcohol in a single word, what would it be and how do you feel about it? This can be serious and thoughtful or fun and silly. For example:

- **Half-dry:** I like keeping my options open, even though I haven't had a drink in six months!

- **DND (Dudes not drinking):** feels cool to not drink.

  Write your own thoughts here!

_____

_____

_____

_____

_____

_____

_____

_____

Letter of Recommendation

IF YOU HAD A VOUCHER—or a few—to give the experience and benefits of going dry to someone else, who would that be? Have you recommended this experience to a friend? A family member? Who else in your inner circle (and outside it) has been impacted or influenced by you going dry?

_____

_____

_____

_____

_____

_____

_____

_____

_____

_____

_____

_____

_____

_____

_____

_____

A Round of Applause!

IT'S FAIR TO SAY YOU'VE ACCOMPLISHED a lot on this journey. And likely learned something, too. What was your proudest moment during this experience? How did this experience change you and/or your vision of going dry (if at all)?

_____

_____

_____

_____

_____

_____

_____

_____

_____

_____

_____

_____

_____

Changing Times

ALONG THE WAY, YOU MAY have thought, "Wow, I would do this differently." Now that you've had time to think about everything, what would you change if you had to do it all again? What was the hardest part of this experience, and what could you do in the future to make it easier?

_____

_____

_____

_____

_____

_____

_____

_____

_____

_____

_____

_____

_____

_____

_____

_____

_____

Back to Buzzy Words

NOW THAT WE'RE NEARING THE END of this book (bittersweet, right?), we're coming full circle. In this exercise, revisit the words in "Buzzy Words" (page 22). This time, circle the words you think of when it comes to going dry. Now that you've experienced it yourself, has your perspective changed?

_____

_____

_____

_____

_____

_____

_____

_____

_____

_____

_____

_____

_____

_____

Note to Self

FOR THE FINAL PROMPT OF THIS BOOK (yay! You made it!), write a letter to your future self. "Future self" can mean the person you envision reading this letter in one month, six months, a year, or even five or ten years down the road. The span of time is up to you. What do you want your future self to know about what you've experienced in the past few months, having made such a big change? Write about any big expectations you had for yourself up to this point. Include any struggles or setbacks you experienced and how you got through them—and/or what they taught you. Also any major milestones and accomplishments you achieved, even if they weren't alcohol related. Final thoughts? Feelings? Notes? Squiggles? Do you have any remaining questions? Get it all out in your letter, sign it, and date it.

Acknowledgments

MANY THANKS TO EVERYONE who ever offered me a drink during the times I was not drinking. Truly (no sarcasm). I've learned so much over the years through questions, trials, awkward moments, and time to reflect in between.

Equally as important: Thank you to the sober community, the kinda-not-drinking right now folks, the Dry/Damp January participants, the abstainer-curious set, and anyone else who has questioned their relationship with alcohol for any amount of time. I am so grateful for your support, friendship, knowledge, and comradery.

Thank you to my incredible editor, Hilary, who obviously is amazing because we have the same name. (Not only that, but she's also great because she edited this book so now you can all read it.) Hilary, thank you for your patience, your feedback, your belief in this workbook, and especially for making this literature 10× more legible. I appreciate you!!!

I'm also very thankful for my agent, Leigh, who asks me pretty regularly what my next book idea is, which is part of the job . . . however, (un?)fortunately for us, this usually spirals into conversations about cakes, cookies, and odd things I've read or observed in the past week. So, thank you, Leigh, for listening to my crazy ideas, and being so kind and patient. And for working with me on another dry book.

Thank you to my family: Matt, Alix, Justin, Nikka, Andrew, Mom and Dad, G and G, and Jim. Dr. and Mrs. L., Kate, Jeff, Leni, Will, Mike, Dave, and Nikki.

And my friends who were especially supportive while writing this: Alyssa, Victoria, Nina, Chelsea, Melissa, Mel, Gab, Amy, Tony, Jaimi, David, Jaclyn and Jon, Jane and Suzie, Sarah and Venessa, Lauryn and Lana, Danielle and Gadi, Tanya, and Katherine and Samantha—who always hold space for me (and usually a nonalcoholic drink, too).

About the Author

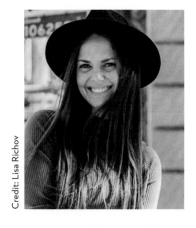

Credit: Lisa Richov

HILARY SHEINBAUM is a journalist and the founder of GoingDry.co. She is also the author of *The Dry Challenge: How to Lose the Booze for Dry January, Sober October, and Any Other Alcohol-Free Month* and a co-author of *A Journal for Bad Days*.

Hilary is a prominent figure in the sober-curious/non-alcoholic beverage space. She is an advocate for dry months and exploring fun, new, and different ways to live a happy, adventurous, big life. She has been featured extensively in news articles and broadcast segments, including MarketWatch's piece on nonalcoholic options on St. Patrick's Day, a front-page story in the *Wall Street Journal,* and a dry dating segment with Michael Strahan on *Good Morning America*. She mixed a NA cocktail on NY1 and discussed Dry January tips on CBS NY, CBS Miami, the *Tamron Hall* show, and NBC Streaming. Hilary also regularly appears on *Good Morning America*'s Instagram and website, making her own NA concoctions. In 2023 *The New York Times* dubbed her "the Dry January M.V.P.," and her first TEDx Talk, covering the topic of dry dating, went live.

The University of Florida graduate started her journalism career as a red carpet reporter, interviewing actors, recording artists, and reality stars. Hilary has contributed to 60+ publications since, including *The New York Times*, the *Wall Street Journal, Bloomberg, USA Today, New York Magazine,* Eater, *HuffPost, Us Weekly, Marie Claire*, and ELLE.com.

Hilary grew up in south Florida, lived long enough in New York to be considered a New Yorker, and often finds herself in Los Angeles (visiting her three brothers).

Resources

Community
The Phoenix: a National Sober Active Community for sober and sober-curious individuals: thephoenix.org

GoingDry.co: public and private non-alcoholic events/experiences and menu curation services: goingdry.co

Recovery
American Addiction Centers*: alcohol.org

Media
Dry Atlas: nonalcoholic beverage news, insights, and recommendations: dryatlas.com

Recovery Rocks Podcast: discussing issues of those who struggle and recover

Zero Proof Nation: a destination for articles and information surrounding nonalcoholic beverages: zeroproofnation.com

*Advice and interactive elements within the text, dry months overall, and dry challenges are not substitutions or replacements for recovery programs. Please speak with your doctor if you are struggling with substances.

Index